MACRONUTRIENT

COOK BOOK

Adaptable diet regimens and delicious recipes for losing weight, building lean muscle

Dorothy M. Hilliard

Table Of Contents

CHAPTER 1

INTRODUCTION

<u>Definition of Macronutrients</u>

Nutrients are chemicals classified into two types: macronutrients and micronutrients. Nutrients are necessary molecules that prevent physiological processes from occurring. Energy provision, structural molecule synthesis, hormone production, and metabolic pathway regulation are all crucial roles provided by macronutrients, which are substances that are required in large quantities. Micronutrients are essential substances that are required at microscopic levels for biochemical processes such as gene transcription regulation, enzyme catalysis, and oxidative stress prevention. Vitamins, minerals, and antioxidants are examples of micronutrients.

The major components of macronutrients are **proteins**, **carbohydrates**, and **lipids**. Alcohol is frequently counted as the fourth macronutrient; nevertheless, alcohol consumption in general is strongly discouraged, and it is not recommended as a source of energy under any circumstances. Although every macronutrient is considered a source of energy, each one has a unique set of biochemical features and has a unique impact on the composition of the body and the individual's health.

The amount of energy contained in each gram (g) of protein, fat, and carbohydrates varies significantly. Throughout this page, kilocalories, abbreviated as kcal, will be referred to as calories.

Carbohydrates

Carbohydrates are an essential source of energy for the diet, and each gram of carbohydrates contains four kilocalories of energy. A higher consumption of carbohydrates causes an increase in blood glucose levels and stimulates insulin secretion, which in turn promotes glucose uptake into tissues and the storage of glucose as glycogen. Additionally, carbohydrates play a significant role in the health of the gut as well as the operation of the immune system. The nondigestible carbohydrate known as fiber, which comes in a variety of subtypes, has a significant role in decreasing cholesterol levels, enhancing gastrointestinal function, and encouraging feelings of fullness in the body.

Proteins

Proteins are huge molecules comprising different numbers and combinations of amino acids connected via peptide bonds. Although dietary proteins contain 4 kcal of energy per gram, they are considered a less efficient energy source than lipids or carbs. Rather, the most significant function of dietary proteins is to provide amino acids, which offer nitrogen, hydrocarbon skeletons, and sulfur. In the human body, amino acids are used for mechanical and structural purposes and help manufacture enzymes, hormones, antibodies, cytokines, transporters, and neurotransmitters. The consumption of dietary protein enhances amino acid availability, stimulates protein synthesis, suppresses protein catabolism, and helps manage whole-body protein balance.

Fats

Lipids, or dietary fats, are the most energy-dense macronutrients and supply 9 kcal of energy per gram. In human physiology, lipids are needed for the generation of sex hormones, preservation of cellular structure, energy storage as body fat, regulation of body temperature, protection from physical harm, as well as fat-soluble vitamins A, D, E, and K. Additionally, fats enhance the taste, texture, and palatability of foods.

Dietary fats can be divided into triglycerides (fats and oils), phospholipids, sterols (cholesterol), and fatty acids. Fatty acids in the diet can be further classified according to the existence of double bonds; saturated fats have no double bonds, and unsaturated fats have one or more double bonds. Finally, unsaturated fatty acids can be separated by the position of the first double bond counted from the methyl end of the carbon chain into omega-3, omega-6, and omega-9 fatty acids, with the first double bond occurring at the third, sixth, and ninth positions, respectively. Different types of dietary lipids have been shown to have distinct physiological features and health implications.

Brief history and popularity

The macrobiotic diet was devised in the 1920s by a Japanese philosopher called George Ohsawa. He felt that by eating a basic, healthful diet, we could live in harmony with nature. He also claimed that his macrobiotic diet could cure cancer and other major disorders.

1970s

The diet became popular in the **1970s**. The term "macrobiotics" refers to a holistic way of eating and living in harmony with nature in order to live a long and healthy life. The premise behind this diet is that a modern western diet is the source of many ailments, such as cancer.

CHAPTER 2
UNDERSTANDING MACRONUTRIENTS

Explanation of Macronutrients

Carbohydrates, protein, and fat are the three macronutrients that comprise food. They provide our bodies, both children and adults, with energy as well as contribute to many other critical body functions.

Most foods contain a combination of the three macronutrients, although foods are generally classified according to which macronutrient they contain the most of.

The main functions are:

Carbohydrates

Carbohydrates, or carbs for short, are our bodies' primary source of energy. They can be found in a variety of foods, including fruits and vegetables, cereals, and dairy products. Carbohydrate-rich foods include: potatoes, rice, pasta, fruit, beans, and oats.

Carbohydrates contain 4 calories per 1g, and the DGA recommends adults get 45–65% of their daily calories from carbs.

Carbohydrates are frequently associated with processed, less nutritious foods such as cookies and white bread. However, many nutritious carbs are the essential basis of a balanced diet. Many of these meals are high in fiber and might help keep you fuller for longer.

Furthermore, carbohydrate energy is critical for fueling the body and brain. The amount of carbs a person needs varies. Some people thrive on lower-carb diets, while others require a diet high in carbs.

Protein

Protein builds and repairs muscle, and other body tissues play an important role in immune function as well as helping transport molecules throughout the body. It can be found in animal foods such as meat, dairy, and eggs, as well as in plant foods like nuts, seeds, whole grains, and soy products. Protein-rich foods include meat, fish, eggs, beans, tofu, and nuts.

There are approximately 4 calories in 1gram of protein. The Dietary Guidelines for Americans (DGA) recommends adults get 10–35% of their daily calories from protein. However, that amount may vary. It varies according to a person's age, body composition objectives, muscle mass, and other factors.

Fats

Fat serves as a long-term source of energy, plays an important role in brain development, and provides insulation and cushioning for the body's organs. Two types of fats, saturated and unsaturated, exist and function differently in the body.

There are 9 calories in 1g of fat. According to the DGA, adults should get 20–35% of their daily calories from fat. Although the diet industry has historically vilified fat, it is essential for a healthy body. Some fats may be a better choice than others. Saturated fats, which are solid at room temperature, should be consumed in moderation by most people. The American Heart Association (AHA) recommends no more than one per day.

Unsaturated fats, such as monounsaturated and polyunsaturated fats, are liquid at room temperature. Nuts, seeds, avocados, and oily fish contain these fats. These are healthy fats, and diets that contain a good amount of these fats have associations with many health benefits. Protein, fat, and carbs all have varying amounts of energy per gram(g). kilocalories (kcal) as simply calories.

Importance of balancing macronutrient intake

For the purpose of maintaining one's health and warding off sickness throughout one's entire life, it is essential to adhere to a nutritious eating pattern that includes nutrient-dense food sources in sufficient quantities. It is necessary for the body to consume a significant amount of macronutrients in order to fulfill its physiologic requirements and maintain its energy needs. Intake of each macronutrient must surpass calorie restrictions while still providing for an acceptable balance between protein, carbs, and fats. This must be accomplished without exceeding the necessary requirements for any macronutrient.

As per the recommendations of the United States Department of Agriculture (USDA), it is recommended that nutrient requirements rather than supplements, be met primarily from entire foods and beverages. This should include a wide variety of foods from various groups, such as fruits, vegetables, legumes, whole grains, nuts, and seeds, while limiting the consumption of added sugars and saturated fats when possible.

Consuming an inadequate amount of macronutrients or an excessive amount of them might have negative impacts on one's health and hence should be avoided.

A particular focus should be placed on avoiding chronic excess calorie consumption as well as weight gain in order to lessen the likelihood of obesity and the illnesses that are connected with it. The optimal consumption of protein should be provided in order to reduce the danger of sarcopenia, particularly in populations that are getting older.

Determine macronutrient ratios

Following the completion of the calculation of their total daily calories, an individual is then able to establish their ratio of macronutrients.

According to the DGA, the following ratio is recommended:

10% to 35% of total calories come from proteins.

Fats: 20–35% of total calories

Carbs: 45–65% of total calories

However, this ratio may not meet everyone's goals. For example, endurance athletes may need more carbs, whereas a person with a metabolic disorder may flourish on a lesser intake of carbs.

CHAPTER 3

BENEFITS OF THE MACRONUTRIENTS

Some reasons why people prefer to count macros include:

1. Meeting weight loss goals
2. Improved athletic performance
3. Managing blood sugar levels

Meeting weight loss goals

With obesity rates on the rise, attempts have been made to describe the function of macronutrient intake in promoting weight gain and supporting weight loss.

Historically, carbohydrates and fats have been considered to be responsible for the increased prevalence of obesity, and low-carbohydrate and low-fat diets have been advocated as possible remedies. However, neither carbohydrates nor fats are inherently fattening, and their limitations have not been demonstrated to be differentially superior in aiding weight loss.

Additionally, it is vital to distinguish between different sources of each macronutrient, as processed versions are connected to weight gain and obesity, while unprocessed forms are not. Because obesity is a complicated illness that comes from excess overall energy consumption rather than any individual macronutrient, emphasizing therapies for macronutrient restriction is unlikely to be beneficial.

Moreover, studies have indicated that public health efforts attempting to limit sugar intake can result in a paradoxical rise in fat consumption. When examining weight loss outcomes, low-fat and low-carbohydrate diets are equally beneficial, similar to other dietary patterns that result in calorie restriction without excluding specific food groups.

Improved athletic performance

Following simple nutrition advice can help boost an athlete's strength, a vital component in many sports. In the nutrition realm, there are three sorts of macronutrients to focus on: carbohydrates, protein, and fats. Let's take a look to see how each of the three macronutrients plays a part in physical performance.

Carbohydrates

Consuming carbs before, during, or after exercise has been demonstrated to help with glycogen synthesis, hormonal modulation, and net muscle protein balance. Although most studies concerning carbs normally focus on before or after exercise, it is crucial to consider taking this macronutrient during as well. This is especially crucial for athletes who exercise for lengthy or frequent bouts throughout the day. Taking in the right amount of carbs can also help modify hormone balance to increase performance.

The hormones insulin and cortisol are primarily affected by carbs in a good way to help move the body into an anabolic stage (a muscle-building state) and enhance protein turnover rate. Taking in carbohydrates before, during, and after exercise can all help maintain muscle protein balance. However, some studies suggest that taking in carbs along with protein may produce the highest gain in net muscle protein balance.

Protein

Protein is a crucial macronutrient utilized to help restore damaged muscular tissue after exercise. Looking into the protein turnover rate is crucial to understanding how nutrition might aid an athlete. When more protein is synthesized than destroyed, more lean muscle mass will be formed, leading to an athlete's exercise performance being boosted.

Supplementing amino acids (protein) is becoming a regular approach to boost workout performance. More precisely, taking in branch chain amino acids (BCAAs) is an appropriate supplement to help maintain the body from catabolizing (breaking down). Not only will this promote muscle protein synthesis, but it will also inhibit intracellular proteolytic pathway activity. In simple words, this means the BCAA's will affect enzyme activity and, therefore, boost protein turnover.

Therefore, with more protein being made and less being broken down, an individual will be able to recover faster and compete for a longer amount of time. Experts have established that the major BCAA, leucine, is the most significant amino acid for proteins. With an increased quantity of muscle mass from a greater protein turnover rate, strength improvements will allow the athlete to compete at a better level throughout their sports.

Lipids (Fats)

It is known that the hormone testosterone has a function in muscle development as well as performance. Fat is arguably the most essential macronutrient to alter testosterone levels in either a favorable or negative way. Since fats are difficult to digest, it's recommended that they not be ingested before or during exercise. Recent research has shown that when fat levels are too low, the hormone balance will begin to severely influence the athlete. Some studies have revealed that optimum fat ratios range from 20–30% of daily calorie intake.

The athlete must also aim to reduce their saturated fats to 10% of their caloric intake. By keeping within these optimal ranges, the athlete will be able to perform at a higher level due to their body's capacity to stay in a more anabolic state because of the elevated testosterone levels. Following these eating rules will enhance exercise performance because of the increased quantity of muscle mass brought on by the body in its anabolic stage. In order to enhance performance, nutrient amount, quality, and timing are all crucial aspects to consider when putting together a nutrition plan for an athlete.

Managing blood sugar levels

This distribution is beneficial for blood sugar management and healthy aging. It has around 40% carbohydrate, 30% protein, and 30% fat. These percentages target blood sugar regulation by increasing protein and lowering the amount of carbohydrates.

CHAPTER 4

HOW TO FOLLOW THE MACRONUTRIENT

Calculating individual macronutrient needs

People should follow several steps before starting a macro diets.

Determine caloric needs

There are a few methods a person might use to figure out their daily calorie needs. First, they can use an internet calculator, such as the popular If It Fits Your Macros (IIFYM) BMR calculator. Using information about a person's health and lifestyle allows the app to estimate a person's daily caloric needs. Additionally, consumers can calculate their calories themselves using a formula.

The Mifflin-St. Jeor equation is a frequent choice:
Men: calories/day = 10 x weight (kg) + 6.25 x height (cm) – 5 x age (y) + 5
Women: calories/day = 10 x weight (kg) + 6.25 x height (cm) – 5 x age (y) – 161

Then, the user doubles their result by an activity factor, which is a figure that represents their daily activity level:
Sedentary: x 1.2 (little or no exercise; desk job)
Lightly active: x 1.375 (mild exercise 1-3 days a week)
Moderately active: x 1.55 (moderate activity 6-7

days a week)

Very active: x 1.725 (hard activity every day or exercise twice a day)

Extra active: x 1.9 (intense workout twice a day or more)

The final value is the person's total daily energy expenditure (TDEE). This is the total quantity of calories they burn per day. People who desire to either lose or gain weight can gently increase or decrease their calories; however, they should do it gradually.

<u>Tracking macronutrients intake</u>

Track macros

After finding the macronutrient ratio, a person needs to log their food. Tracking macros entails tracking the foods ingested and paying attention to the macronutrients taken.

There are a few techniques to track macros. For many people, the easiest way is to use a website or smartphone app. Others prefer to do the math by hand, although this takes more time. This often entails a person determining how many grams of each macronutrient they will take each day by applying the following formula: (Total daily calories x macronutrient%) / calories per gram So, if a person eating 2,000 calories per day wanted to know how many grams of carbs they should consume and they desired to receive 50% of their daily consumption from carbs, they would calculate:

(2,000 x 0.50) / 4 = 250g carbohydrate

Meal and planning and food choices

A macro diet entails counting the intake of three macronutrients: proteins, lipids, and carbs. First, a person works out their daily calorie needs, then they split the calories into proportions, such as **10–35% proteins, 20–35% fats, and 45–65% carbs.**

While all foods are allowed, it's easier to fulfill your macro-objectives with a diet rich in fruits, vegetables, high-quality proteins, nuts, seeds, and whole grains.

CHAPTER 5

SAMPLE MACRONUTRIENTS WEIGHT LOSS MEAL PLAN

There is no single optimum food plan for weight loss. However, adopting a diet rich in natural foods and reducing processed foods is an excellent starting point. This describes how to plan a meal for weight loss and gives a 7-day meal plan to consider and employ other beneficial techniques for weight loss for different groups and people with varying dietary restrictions.

How to plan meals for weight loss

A person should plan their meals according to their requirements. They should consider

- How much weight they need to lose
- Their activity levels
- Any dietary requirements for health conditions
- Any personal, cultural, or religious dietary requirements
- How much available time they have for food preparation and shopping
- Their level of cooking expertise and the difficulty of recipes
- Whether the meal plan needs to include other members of the household.

The following section contains a healthy meal plan for weight loss that a person can adapt as necessary.

7-day weight loss meal plans with grocery list

The following meal plan includes options for 7 days of meals and snacks. The plan comprises nutrient-dense whole foods.A person should identify the optimal portion sizes according to their weight loss objectives, activity levels, and specific requirements.

Day	Breakfast	Lunch	Dinner	Snacks
1	scrambled egg with spinach and tomato	tuna salad with lettuce, cucumber, and tomato	bean chili with cauliflower 'rice'	apple slices and peanut butter
2	oatmeal with	hummus and	sesame salmon,	tangerine and

	blueberries, milk, and seeds	vegetable wrap	purple sprouting broccoli, and sweet potato mash	cashew nuts
3	mashed avocado and a fried egg on a slice of rye toast	broccoli quinoa and toasted almonds	chicken stir fry and soba noodles	blueberries and coconut yogurt

4	smoothie made with protein powder, berries, and oat milk	chicken salad with lettuce and corn	roasted Mediterranean vegetables, puy lentils, and tahini dressing	whole grain rice cake with nut butter
5	buckwheat pancakes with raspberries and Greek	vegetable soup with two oatcakes	fish tacos with slaw	boiled egg with pita slices

	yogurt			
6	apple slices with peanut butter	minted pea and feta omelet	baked sweet potato, chicken breast, greens	cocoa protein ball
7	breakfast muffin with eggs and vegetables	crispy tofu bowl	lentil Bolognese with zucchini noodles	carrot sticks and hummus

A weight-loss diet plan might sometimes begin at the grocery store. Planning ahead might help when it comes to shopping and consuming the correct foods. If a person can envision their shelves and refrigerator full of nutritious items, they may also be less motivated to add bad variety to their supply.

A person can consider the following tips: Creating a meal plan for the week ahead includes nutritious meals and basing a grocery list exclusively on what those meals need. Then, resolve to purchase only what is on the list to avoid choosing unhealthy snacks.

Visualizing the store layout ahead and avoiding the ice cream and confectionery aisles to limit temptation.

Reducing trips to the grocery shop by stocking up on healthful goods that are easy to store, such as lentils, oats, quinoa, and rice. Order groceries for collection to avoid temptation when strolling past the baked goods aisle.

Healthy additions to add to any grocery list include:

- Canned or dried beans and lentils
- Grains, such as brown rice and quinoa
- Fresh and frozen fruits and vegetables

Fish and lean meats, including turkey

- Eggs
- Yogurt
- Oatmeal

Understanding exactly what is required and avoiding foods high in added sugar and fat can make grocery shopping easier.

Weight reduction and meal plans for vegetarians and vegans

When evaluating how to lose weight, vegetarians and vegans should include nutritious meals and restrict refined carbs and processed foods. People should pay careful attention to packaging labels when choosing meat alternatives, as many of these items have additional sugar and fat.

People who adopt a plant-based diet will also need to ensure that their meals contain enough protein. Some good sources of plant protein include:

- Soy

- Nuts
- Beans
- Whole grains
- Vegan meal plan

Research reveals that those who adopt a vegan diet are likely to have a lower body mass index (BMI) compared to omnivore diets and pescatarian   diets.

Vegan diets are fully plant-based, which means they do not include meat, eggs, or dairy products.

Vegan diets omit several foods heavy in fat, cholesterol, calories, and saturated fat. However, since animal diets contain vitamin B12, people adopting a vegan diet will need to find alternate sources of B12, such as supplements or fortified plant milks and cereals.

The following is an example of a 1-day vegan meal plan.

Breakfast

Oatmeal with one-quarter cup of cooked rolled oats, a half cup of sliced banana, one-quarter cup of peanut butter, and soy or almond milk.

Lunch

Grain bowl with 1 cup of quinoa and 1 cup of mixed vegetables, including chick peas, Brussels sprouts, and broccoli.

Dinner

Sweet potato tacos with avocado, onion, and tomato

Snack

Hummus with carrot and celery sticks

Vegetarian meal plan

Those who adopt a vegetarian diet eschew meat and fish but may continue to eat eggs and dairy products.

Research indicates that following a vegetarian diet can be an efficient way to lose weight.

However, people who adopt a vegetarian diet need to be careful about what they eat to ensure they achieve their nutritional requirements.

The below meal plan provides an example of what one day following a vegetarian diet may contain

Breakfast

2 hard-boiled eggs with a dash of hot sauce and salt

Lunch

Kale salad with raisins, chickpeas, walnuts, and roasted sweet potatoes

Dinner

Black bean burgers with avocado and roasted Brussels sprouts on the side

Snack

Plain yogurt with granola

<u>**Weight loss meal plan for people with diabetes**</u>

Losing weight can help a person with diabetes maintain their blood sugar levels and avoid complications.

According to the American Diabetes Association, patients with diabetes should reduce weight by a mix of exercise, diet, and portion control. Low glycemic index (GI) foods can help someone avoid increases in blood sugar while they lose weight.

A person who has type 1 diabetes should visit their doctor or nutritionist for help establishing a weight loss strategy. People will need to regulate their food to work alongside any drugs they take to control their blood sugar levels.

Diabetes meal plan

For those with diabetes, a healthy meal plan should focus on whole foods rather than processed foods to help manage blood sugar levels as much as possible. It will include non-starchy veggies such as broccoli, spinach, and green beans. It will also integrate fewer added sugars and processed carbs, such as white bread, rice, or pasta.

Below is an illustration of what one day following a diabetes meal plan may include:

Breakfast

2-egg omelet with vegetables (spinach, mushrooms, bell pepper, avocado), and 1 cup blueberries on the side.

Lunch

Sandwich: 2 regular slices high fiber whole grain bread, 2 oz canned tuna in water mixed with 1 tbsp lemon juice, and 1 mashed avocado

Dinner

1 cup cooked lentil penne pasta, 1.5 cups veggie tomato sauce (cook garlic, mushrooms, greens, zucchini, and eggplant into it), 2 oz ground lean turkey

Snack

15–20 baby carrots with 2 tbsp plain hummus

Heart-healthy weight loss and meal plan

Dietary decisions can contribute to obesity and type 2 diabetes, which can increase a person's risk of cardiovascular disease. A heart-healthy meal plan includes meals that boost cardiovascular benefits, such as vegetables, whole grains, and oily salmon. It also prohibits red and processed meats, alcohol, and foods high in sugar and salt.Examples of heart-healthy diets include the Dietary Approaches to Stop Hypertension (DASH) diet, the Mediterranean diet, and vegetarian diets. Research from a trusted source demonstrates all of these diets can help reduce cardiovascular disease.Below are some meal ideas for a heart-healthy diet.

Heart-healthy meal plans

Breakfast

Mixed fruit parfait (cantaloupe, strawberries, blueberries, kiwi) with a side of whole grain toast

Lunch

1 cup whole grain pasta with mixed vegetables (tomato, onion, kale) cooked in a skillet with 1 tbsp lemon and olive oil

Dinner

2 serving of salmon, with a side of green beans

Snacks

1 cup of mixed nuts — almonds, walnuts, and cashews

Approaches for other groups

Dietary requirements vary. There are a number of techniques for weight loss that may suit various people.

A 2017 systematic review studied the

effectiveness of weight loss programs in males. The review indicated that the following measures were the most successful for facilitating weight loss:

- A calorie-restricted diet
- Physical activity advice
- And an activity and behavior-change program

However, while this review looked mainly at measures for guys, these tactics work for girls too.

The review also reveals that participants preferred face-based language and personal feedback.

People who want this type of support and counsel may benefit from using applications such as My Fitness Pal or seeking aid from a personal trainer or licensed dietician. Weight loss with pregnancy and breastfeeding. Dieting during pregnancy and breastfeeding may not be appropriate. Anyone concerned about their weight or general fitness during pregnancy or nursing should contact a doctor or midwife for further guidance.

Weight loss and menopause

People going through menopause may find it more difficult to lose weight. A 2019 study found that fat mass and body weight tend to increase throughout the menopause transition. The study indicated that the women had an average fat mass increase of 1–1.7% per year of the transition, resulting in a 6% overall gain in fat mass across the 3.5-year transition period.

The average weight increase among the individuals was 1.6 kilos.

Females who seek to reduce weight during menopause should ensure that they consume adequate nutrients to support their bone health. **Nutrients include:**

Vitamin D, calcium Vitamin K, magnesium

How many calories to lose weight? According to the National Heart, Lung, and Blood Institute (NHLBI), to reduce weight successfully and securely, people should aim to drop 1-2 pounds each week for 6 months. A person can accomplish this degree of weight loss by cutting their calorie consumption by 500–1,000 calories each day.

However, the body can also create hormonal changes when a person decreases their calorie intake, and their weight reduction may plateau as a result.

Many low-calorie diets restrict fats; however, fats help a person feel full. As such, some people may not be able to sustain a low-fat diet.

People should also remember that calorie reduction alone may not be sufficient for maintaining weight loss. This is because foods with the same amount of calories might have varied impacts on a person's metabolism.

For example, high-GI foods could have harmful consequences for a person's weight loss goals.

According to a 2014 randomized controlled trials, the following foods could cause:

- Rises in blood glucose levels and insulin levels, cravings for high-carbohydrate foods
- Increased fat storage

Some examples of high-GI foods include:

- Sugary foods
- Sweet soft drinks
- White bread, white rice, and potatoes

In addition to lowering calories and eating healthy meals, individuals may wish to consider integrating an exercise regimen to support their weight loss objectives.

A 2020 study comparing diet against a diet and exercise program for health enhancement and weight loss among overweight women aged 40–60 years indicated that a combination diet and exercise approach had the best effects. Evaluated the ideal nutritional regimen for effective and sustainable weight loss among adults who were overweight or obese. The review found that there is no single fit-for-all diet and that the optimum strategy is individualization. **The same review underlines the usefulness of the following approaches for weight loss:**

- Avoiding added sugars
- Limiting processed foods
- Ingesting full-grain products
- Eating more fruit and veggies

Other weight loss tips

Alongside meal planning and following a shopping list, some other strategies that may help a person lose weight include:

- Being cognizant of portion size and the ratios of different macronutrients, including protein and fiber, in every meal.

- Exploring different herbs and spices to add diversity to meals and decreasing the need for excessive sugar, salt, and fat.

- Cooking nutritious meals for the freezer avoiding lengthy periods without eating to minimize cravings for unhealthy snacks.

- Keeping hydrated to lessen cravings for sugary drinks.

- Performing 30 minutes moderate-intensity physical activity on most or all days of the week, partnering with a diet and exercise buddy using weighing scales no more than once a week at a regular hour of the day.

Summary

Combining a nutritious diet with an active lifestyle can help a person maintain a reasonable weight. Planning meals and shopping is beneficial for healthy weight loss.

Counting calories may not be the sole beneficial technique for weight loss. A weight loss program is more successful when a person modifies it to their specific requirements.

A registered dietitian or certified nutrition specialist can assist a person in developing an ideal meal plan and support the person while working toward their weight loss objectives.

CHAPTER 6

TIPS FOR SUCCESS ON THE MACRONUTRIENTS

<u>Staying consistent with tracking</u>

The number one thing we try to do with people who are either new to tracking or have a hectic lifestyle is to pre-plan your macros for the next day.

So, when you're sitting on the sofa at night watching TV or perusing Instagram, use that time to also input your food for the next day, so you're prepared and less likely to miss your numbers. No more standing in the kitchen wasting time trying to figure out what you're going to eat, either!

We seldom see anyone miss their macros when they have their day already mapped out in MFP or whatever program they're using. It sucks when you get to the end of the day and you feel like you can't get to your goals, but we can't have such high expectations for results when we aren't matching our efforts to them. But just one tiny job of pre-planning your macros can make all the difference. Plus, it takes all   of   10   minutes!

<u>**A Step-by-Step Guide to Staying Consistent With Tracking Macros**</u>

These are the steps we offer to customers and follow ourselves to get to the point where you're removing the guesswork out of tracking macros and hitting them with ease on a day-to-day basis. It might sound like a bold claim for us to state that it will be easy for you to hit macros someday, but if you spend the time following these methods, you will get there.

STEP 1:

PLAN OUT A FULL DAY OF FOOD WITH EASY-TO-TRACK AND SIMPLE MEALS THAT FIT YOUR MACROS.

If you are new to macros, trying something more sophisticated, like a meal with a ton of components, can be frustrating. You can accomplish this eventually, but it can get confusing and time-consuming. When you are cooking for numerous people, set something aside for you and continue to cook for others as you usually would. It won't be like this forever, but for the sake of learning how to track at the beginning, this will make things less complicated.

TIP: Evenly distribute your macros throughout the day. The best method to do this is to take your macros and divide them by the number of meals you intend to consume that day, and use those as your target macros for each meal. Example: You have 100 grams of protein and plan to have 4 meals—that's 25 grams of protein per meal. Do the same for your carbs and fats!

STEP 2:

EAT THE SAME MEALS FOR 2-21 DAYS
Yes, this sounds like a vast range, but this is going to be very person-dependent. If you're someone who's been tracking for a little while and is having a hard time resetting, you might not need as many days. If you're newer, you might need to do this for longer, maybe even a month.

Now, this is temporary until you get a better handle on pre-planning and hitting your meals each day. The more you do this, the more it will feel like a habit or routine to do so, and you'll be more comfortable mixing up your meals utilizing the same macronutrient breakdown for your   meals.

STEP 3:

LEARN HOW TO COOK BASIC FOODS (SO THEY ACTUALLY TASTE GOOD)
Many folks choke down their "healthy" food or don't eat it at all since they aren't enjoying their meals.

This is where we'd like to remind you not to underestimate the power of seasonings and condiments! They genuinely influence how tasty a dish is, especially when it comes to preparing chicken, ground turkey or beef, rice, fish, vegetables,   etc.

Step 4:

ALWAYS HAVE PLAN MOVING FORWARD

You've heard it before: "Failing to plan is planning to fail." We cannot hammer that home enough. If you don't know what the day holds, develop a loose plan with what you can and make preparations for everything that comes up. It's going to happen, so use it as a learning opportunity.

Step 5:

TRACK WITH EASE

Now you have a base for how to navigate counting macros consistently!

CONCLUSION

A recap of the macronutrients and their benefits

Macronutrients are the nutrients that your body needs in significant amounts, which include fat, carbs, and protein. They're the nutrients that give you energy and are commonly dubbed "macros." Macronutrients contain the components of food that your body needs to maintain its systems and structures.

Encouragement for readers to try macronutrients

As a general guideline, macronutrient breakdown is 20%–30% fat, 30% protein, and 40%–50% carbs." Focus on consuming healthy fats from items like nuts, seeds, olive oil, salmon, and avocados, with portion control in mind, because fats are higher in calories.

www.ingramcontent.com/pod-product-compliance
Lightning Source LLC
Chambersburg PA
CBHW071101260726
48661CB00006B/2381